Table of Contents

Introduction

I want to thank you and congratulate you for downloading the book, The Fatty Liver and Weight Loss Solution, Proven Natural, Safe and Non-Toxic Strategies to Reverse, Cure and Prevent Fatty Liver.

Fatty liver is a precursor to a more serious disease- liver failure. Stop and reverse this condition in its early stages to reduce mortality and morbidity, with just a simple change in diet and lifestyle.

Read on and learn just how you can promote better liver health for a better and healthier body.

Thanks again for downloading this book. I hope you enjoy it!

Chapter 1 Knowing the Liver

One of the body's vital organs is the liver. Food nutrients right from the intestines are processed within the liver. It binds, unbinds, remodels and restructures molecules to render them active or inactive, for circulation or for excretion. And because it handles one of the body's "dirty jobs", it, too cannot escape damage from too much toxins.

Anatomy of the liver

Weighing on an average of 3 pounds, the liver is the second largest organ in the body, next to the skin. Of all internal organs, this is the largest. It has a reddish-brown color, with a rubbery texture. The entire organ is encapsulated by a tough fibrous tissue, further reinforced by the peritoneum. The peritoneal layer both covers and keeps the liver in its place in the abdominal cavity. The liver is protected by the lower portion of the rib cage.

Two large sections comprise the liver- a right and a left lobe. Most of the mass is concentrated in the right lobe. This portion descends downwards into the abdominal cavity.

Blood supply comes from two large blood vessels. The portal vein brings blood into the liver from the digestive tract, bringing with it nutrients for metabolism, restructuring and repackaging for storage, activation, inactivation or excretion. The hepatic artery brings nourishing blood into the liver from the heart.

Location

The main body of the liver is located in the right upper quadrant of the abdominal cavity. It lies underneath the diaphragm. The lower portion of the rib cage provides the most protection for the liver against external trauma.

The upper part of the liver extends across the middle of the abdomen towards the left upper quadrant. When the liver enlarges (such as in inflammation and disease conditions), part of it extends downwards to the umbilical area and the upper portion extends further across the upper abdominal area.

One incredible thing about the liver is its capacity to repair and regenerate dead and damaged tissues. It can accelerate the rate of cellular division in order to restore the liver's size and, ultimately, its function.

Functioning Liver

The liver has many functions, from digestion to immunity.

Digestive function

Bile plays a major role in digestion and it is produced by hepatocytes in the liver. It is composed of cholesterol, salts, water and bilirubin. It functions as an emulsifier for fat digestion. Fat is difficult to digest because of its oily nature. With the help of bile, it coats the surfaces of fat molecules, making them more responsive to digestive enzymes.

Red Blood Cells (RBC) Processing

The liver digests old and worn out red blood cells. When the blood flows into the liver, the Kupffer cells filter out any old red blood cells and pass them on to the hepatocytes. The hemoglobin in RBC is separated into its different units, the heme and the globin. Heme is the iron-containing group that can no longer be recycled by the body. It is converted into bilirubin, which is added to the bile. It gives the characteristic greenish color of the bile. Bilirubin separates from the bile once it is the intestines. Bacteria in the intestines act upon bilirubin to convert it into stercobilin, the compound that gives the brownish color of feces. The globin portion is recycled by the liver into separate components and used as energy.

Carbohydrate Metabolism

Blood from the digestive system carries with it the broken down particles of the different nutrients such as monosaccharide glucose. The hepatocytes take glucose, restructure them and store them in the form of glycogen. This stored glycogen is structured in such a way that the liver can store large amounts of it and ne able to release them fast enough whenever the serum glucose levels drop. The conversion of glucose into glycogen protects the body from harmful spikes and sudden drops in the blood sugar levels. This process also maintains homeostasis.

Fat Metabolism

Digested fats are absorbed by lacteals- special blood vessels designed to carry fatty acids into the liver. In its raw, just-digested form, fatty acids cannot enter the blood vessels because of its oily nature and naturally large molecules. These are brought to the liver so that the hepatocytes can restructure them and enable them to join the bloodstream.

Fatty acids are modified to form lipids that the body can use. They are attached to several proteins to form VLDL (very low density lipoprotein), LDL (low density lipoprotein), HDL (high density lipoprotein, triglycerides, phospholipids, lipoproteins and cholesterol. Proteins act as carrier proteins that enable the blood to pick up the fats and bring them to the cells for use and storage.

The liver is also responsible for how much of the fats get into the blood for circulation and how much to be excreted. It all depends on what protein the liver attaches to the fatty acids. Should the fatty acid be tagged for excretion, it joins the bile and enters to the intestines for elimination via the feces.

Protein Metabolism

Proteins in food are broken down into amino acids through digestion. As it is, the body cannot use raw, newly digested amino acids. They need to be restructured and tagged in order to fit into the receptor sites on the body's cell surfaces. This process happens, where else, in the liver.

Hepatocytes in the liver remove the amine groups, convert them into ammonia and then to urea. The urea reenters the blood and goes to the kidney for excretion. The other components of amino acids are further broken down by the hepatocytes to form ATP or new glucose molecules for storage.

Storage

The liver stores many of the body's absorbed essential vitamins, nutrients and minerals. It stores carbohydrates, fats and proteins from digested materials by converting them into glycogen.

Also, the liver stores fat-soluble vitamins like vitamins A, D, E and K, and vitamin B12. Minerals like copper and iron are also stored in the liver. The storage allows a steady supply of these essential nutrients to the tissues of the body.

Detoxification

Most of the toxins in the blood enter through the digestive system. It metabolizes toxins and renders them inactive and structured for excretion.

Protein synthesis

Proteins important for clotting like fibrinogen and prothrombin are manufactured in the liver. These are important for clot formation to stop bleeding and promote healing of injured tissues.

Another important protein is albumin. It is a plasma protein that plays an important role in keeping the isotonic environment of the blood plasma. This crucial balance needs to be maintained in order for other compounds, hormones, electrolytes and enzymes will be effectively transported to their respective sites of action.

Immunity

The Kupffer cells in the liver tissues are fixed macrophages, playing a part in the mononuclear phagocyte system. It works in coordination with the macrophages found in the lymph nodes and spleen.

These special cells capture nay bacteria circulating along with the blood. It also digests parasites and fungi, as well as cellular debris and old, worn-out red blood cells.

Chapter 2 Fatty Liver- Risk Factors, Causes & Symptoms

Also known as steatosis, fatty liver disease refers to the buildup of excessive fatty deposits within the liver cells. This is the most common complaint that involves this large internal organ. Statistics show that 1 in every 10 people suffer from fatty liver disease.

The liver normally has fat deposits within its structure, so are all the other body organs. What makes it of concern is its excessive amounts. Too much fatty buildup in the liver interferes with its normal functioning. Too much means if the fat is more than 10% of the liver's weight.

Fatty liver stimulates an inflammatory reaction. The immune system sends cells to destroy the source of irritation (i.e., the excess fats). The healthy liver cells become collateral damage to the inflammatory process. Because of the liver's amazing ability for cell repair and regeneration, fatty liver, in itself is a reversible and self-limiting, meaning- it heals on its own.

However, if the damage is extensive, and the excess fatty deposits keep on accumulating, the liver will find it difficult to catch up. It will double its efforts at repairing the damage. The result, however, is the production of too many scarred and hardened tissues. When this happens, the condition is now considered as liver cirrhosis.

Causes

The main cause of having fatty liver is eating too much calories. The liver stores a lot of the unused calories within its structure, creating a growing layer of fat.

Another major cause of fatty liver is alcoholism- too much intake of alcohol. When a person drinks too much alcohol, say, in excess of the recommended 1-2 drinks per day, the liver is on the protective mode. Alcohol, in high amounts, is considered as a toxin in the body. It goes straight to the liver. The liver responds to the offending substance by protecting itself from the damaging effect. It converts all available nutrients in the blood into fats, in an attempt to from a protective fatty layer. Most people who tested for fatty liver have been found to have either recently consumed large amounts or are chronic heavy alcohol drinkers.

Fatty liver may be a result of other diseases like:

- diabetes
- metabolic disorders
- metabolic syndrome X
- high blood cholesterol
- excess body weight
- insulin resistance (type 2 diabetes)
- high levels of triglycerides (fats) in the blood

It may also be brought about intake of certain medications like:

- aspirin
- steroids
- tamoxifen
- tetracycline
- Other causes include:
- pregnancy
- toxins
- viruses (hepatitis A, etc.)

Risk Factors

Statistics show that most people diagnosed with fatty liver are overweight and middle-aged.

- Overweight with BMI between 25 to 30
- Obesity with BMI of more than 30
- Diabetes
- High levels of triglycerides

Other risk factors

- Too much alcohol use

- Too much use of OTC like NSAIDs
- Type 2 diabetes
- Pregnancy
- High cholesterol levels
- Elevated triglyceride levels
- Malnutrition
- Metabolic syndrome

Symptoms

Usually, fatty liver has no symptoms. The liver constantly repairs and regenerates damaged cells, so that there may be little to no symptoms. The following are some of the most common indications that the liver may be suffering from too much fatty deposits:

- Jaundice (yellowing of the skin)
- Fatigue
- Nausea
- Vomiting

Types

Acute Fatty Liver Related to Pregnancy

This rare form of fatty liver can be life threatening. The symptoms start to be felt by the 3rd trimester of pregnancy. Symptoms include vomiting, nausea, jaundice, pain over the upper right quadrant of the abdomen and general malaise. This condition improves without any further medical treatment after delivery.

Nonalcoholic Fatty Liver

This type develops because the liver has difficulty metabolizing fats that leads to buildup within the tissues of the liver. Alcohol has no direct hand in the development of this type of fatty liver. This type is actually very common and most often linked to overweight and obesity conditions.

This type has four stages. While it often goes away on its own, it has the possibility of progressing into a more serious liver problem.

Simple fatty liver

Also called hepatic steatosis. This stage is characterized by excess amounts of fats accumulating in the liver cells. Most people experience no symptoms. In some, it can progress to more serious forms.

Non Alcoholic Steatohepatitis

The accumulation of too much fat in the liver produces inflammatory reaction. Liver cell damage start to occur.

Fibrosis

Persistent inflammation of the liver results to the formation of scar tissues. The scar tissues are called fibrosis. A few fibrotic tissues do not significantly impair the liver function. Large or too many scar tissues can cause a significant decline in the functioning of the liver.

Cirrhosis

This condition describes a liver that is full of fibrotic tissues. Functioning is significantly impaired, which can often lead to live failure.

Risk Factors for Non Alcoholic Fatty Liver Disease (NAFLD)

Obesity

Studies have found that most people diagnosed with NAFLD are overweight or obese. However, the exact mechanism of how obesity and overweight causes fatty liver is still unknown. It has actually been found that mildly overweight people have a higher risk of developing fatty liver than very obese people.

Diabetes

People with type 2 diabetes have a higher risk of developing fatty liver than those with type 2 diabetes mellitus. The idea is that the fatty accumulation has something to do with impaired insulin function and regulation. Insulin triggers the fat storage, and impaired insulin action causes more fats to deposit within the liver cells.

Age

Advancing age increases the possibility of developing fatty liver. It is believed that the body loses its ability to effectively metabolize and store nutrients, leading to fat accumulation within the structure of the liver. Statistics show that NAFLD occurs more often among people who are more than 50 years of age.

High blood pressure

People with high blood pressure have a higher risk for NAFLD. Hypertension is already associated with elevated cholesterol levels, which contributes to fatty buildup in the liver.

Hyperlipidemia

High amount of fats in the blood is called hyperlipidemia. This is particularly high cholesterol and triglyceride levels.

Weight loss

Losing weight at a very rapid rate increases the risk for fatty liver disease. The fats and fatty acid amounts in the blood change rapidly and the body feels threatened by it. The response is to store more fat, which increases the risk for fatty liver development. Also, people who underwent surgical intervention for obesity (i.e., bariatric surgery) have been found to develop NAFLD after the surgery.

Medications

Some medications are very toxic to the liver, like tamoxifen. Chronic use of drugs like NSAIDs can cause toxic buildup of chemicals in the blood, which threatens the liver. In response to the threats of cellular damage from these medications, the liver increases its rate of fat conversion and storage to provide a protective pad around its structure.

Symptoms of NAFLD

Generally, fatty liver does not cause any symptoms. But in some people, and when the disease becomes more serious, NAFLD can cause the following:

- Persistent pain over the upper right portion of the abdomen, where the liver is located
- Enlarged liver, felt upon palpation
- Easily gets tired

Alcoholic Fatty Liver Disease

This form of fatty liver is a direct result of alcohol consumption. Alcohol is toxic to the body in large amounts. Fatty liver while taking alcohol is a warning sign that alcohol consumption is already at an alarmingly dangerous level.

Usually, fatty liver related to alcohol consumption reverses naturally if the person stops drinking alcohol.

Millions of people worldwide drink a lot of alcohol. Most of the people who abuse alcohol develop fatty livers, almost 90 to 100% actually. Fat accumulation can occur even a short while after consuming large amounts of alcohol. Take note that safe alcohol amounts is only 1 to 2 glasses of wine, or 1 to 2 bottles of beer, or 1 shot of distilled spirits. More than any of this (not all or combination) is already considered high level of consumption and trigger fat accumulation.

Having alcoholic fatty liver is actually the first stage of liver disease related to alcoholism. The liver becomes damaged by alcohol, which impairs its ability to breakdown fats. Continuing on this path will result in too much damage, leading to widespread scarring and fibrotic tissue development. When this occurs, liver cirrhosis and eventually, liver failure will develop.

Chapter 3 Weight Loss for Treatment

Obesity is one of the main reasons for fatty liver development. Losing weight helps in preventing, as well as treatment for fatty liver. By reducing the amount of fat in the body, little by little, the body starts to metabolize the excess fats in the liver until it all but disappears.

Lose weight slowly

Losing weight is the most effective and the mandatory method to stop fatty buildup and reverse fatty liver disease. There are no medical treatments for fatty liver, and if the liver cannot adequately keep its rate of repair to the rate of fatty buildup, it may progress to the more serious cirrhosis.

By losing weight, the fatty buildup is slowly burned. The body loses or uses much of the stored fat. Overweight or obese, losing weight is absolutely the first on the list for fatty liver reversal.

Safe weight loss is done by losing just about 1 to 2 pounds per week. Studies on weight loss to treat or relieve fatty liver showed that the condition significantly improves by losing at least 9% of the total body weight. The weight loss should be spread over a period of months, not in mere days, as in crash dieting and excessive exercise. Another study also found out that even if the weight loss is less than 9%, fatty buildup in the liver is significantly slowed.

Studies have shown that losing much weight too rapidly can actually cause more harm to the liver. The body recognizes rapid weight loss as starvation. The body reacts by conserving all available nutrients and actually increases the rate of storage. The body is designed to be on the protective mode if conditions indicate any threat to survival. The liver speeds up its rate of fat storage and invariably reduces the rate of fat burning. The result of rapid weight loss is more fat storage, making the condition worse than before.

Lifestyle Changes for Weight Loss

Making healthier changes in the lifestyle is a slower but safer and more sustainable weight loss method. Crash diets do help in losing weight but will only be effective during the first week. Beyond that, the body will start to feel threatened and will go on conservation mode. If the body loses weight gradually, it has enough time to adjust to the slowly decreasing food intake and lifestyle change.

Before starting on weight loss, get the present weight and calculate how much should be lost. Generally, minimum weight loss is at 10%. Best to consult with the doctor in deciding exactly how much weight should be lost.

Next step is to plan how to lose the weight. It isn't all about weight machine and long sweaty hours in the gym. A few simple changes in the choices you make each day can already help in reducing weight.

- Taking the stairs for the last couple of floors.

- Choose to park farther from the entrance the next time you go shopping.

- Do your grocery shopping while on a full stomach. You may be surprised. You will be less tempted to buy food, no matter how tempting they look. Your mind will be dwelling on the fact that you are already full, hence, less interest in food.

- Saying no to desserts. Make it a rule to have dessert only during special occasions.

- Snack on fresh fruits and vegetables instead of chips and candies. Munch on carrot sticks and cucumber slices whenever you feel you need a snack, an energy boost or you feel you want to munch on something. Always a batch already washed, peeled and sliced in the refrigerator or in small carry snack boxes.

- Infused water, sugar-free is better than drinking soft drinks with high amounts of fructose.

- Brisk walking each day for 30 minutes helps in steady, continuous weight loss. Good for the heart, too.

- Choose leaner, healthier sources of proteins like white meat in turkey and chicken- without the skin on.

- Avoid foods with high glycemic index. Choose healthier foods.

- Water. Lots of it. Stay hydrated. The body often mistakes thirst for feelings of hunger.

Chapter 4 Dietary Means of Treatment

Diet helps reverse fatty liver disease. By reducing the amount of fat that enters the body, the fat in the liver has a chance to be metabolized and turned into usable fats.

Dietary changes aim to reduce the amount of fat deposited within the structure of the liver and minimize the damage to the liver cells. The food choices are also focused on improving the function of insulin. This hormone plays a major role in the conversion of carbohydrates into fats. Also, making better food choices helps in losing weight faster, which is the main option for improving fatty liver conditions.

Studies have shown that even if a person has trouble losing weight, changing the diet can significantly help improve fatty liver conditions.

To start, remove or at least reduce to a minimum the amount of sugar, fat, cholesterol and empty calories. You will amazed by how much good this will do to the body- better lipid profile, better health, better sugar control, to name a few.

What to avoid

Fructose

This is a very common ingredient in most foods today. It can be found in products like processed fruit juices, tomato sauce, salad dressings, ketchup- just to name a few. They are found in a wide range of products, so you need to read labels to identify those that have been made with fructose. It is usually labeled as high fructose corn syrup.

Fructose is a very concentrated form of sugar. Just think- a serving of store-bought tomato sauce has more sugar content than a serving of Oreo cookies. You are depriving yourself of sweet treats in place of something that is actually more unhealthy.

White, processed, refined flour

Like fructose, refined, white or processed flour is a very common ingredient in most foods. Even the seemingly healthy whole grain flours pose a problem. They still have undergone some refinement process, which makes the starch they contain a potential health hazard. To be sure, avoid anything that has undergone food processing- no matter how small the processing might have been.

Partially Hydrogenated vegetable oils

This type of oil is the unhealthiest of all oils. Partially hydrogenated oils are also known as trans fat. Don't be fooled by huge prints of "Zero Trans Fat" but has partially hydrogenated oils listed at the back in small print.

This type of oil is damaging to the liver, because of its structure. The body cannot metabolize partially hydrogenated fat, yet it can manipulate the cellular membranes and damage cells.

Other Unhealthy Fats

Aside from trans fat (partially hydrogenated fat), fats bad for the body include fatty meats and preserved mats, suet, lard and drippings.

Foods with high glycemic index

A study conducted in 2007 show that a diet rich in foods with high glycemic index leads to fatty liver. Over the course of 6 months, the liver had twice the amount of fat in its structure than at the start of the study while on a diet with high glycemic foods.

The starch in this type of food is quickly digested and converted into glucose, resulting in sugar spikes. In response, the liver secretes high levels of insulin to quickly store the excess sugar. Stored sugar becomes fatty deposits.

Foods high in glycemic index include:

- Anything made with white, refined or processed lour like white breads and bagels
- Breakfast cereals like instant oatmeal, puffed rice, corn flakes and bran flakes
- White rice
- Rice cakes and rice pasta
- Saltine crackers and pretzels
- Pumpkin, white potato and Russet potato

What to eat

Fats and oils from healthy sources

Oils from fatty fishes like tuna and salmon are rich in omega-3 fatty acids. This king of healthy essential fat reduces the inflammation in the body. By reducing inflammation, the repair of damaged liver speeds up. Less damage also results from this liver problem. Good sources include mackerel, salmon, trout, albacore tuna, sardines, and herring, to name a few.

Another good source is vegetable oils. They contain healthy monounsaturated fats, which the body actually needs for its various processes. Cold pressed oils are good for the body. Heated oils are restructured and cause damage to the cells. Healthy oils include coconut butter, olive oil, and macadamia nut oils.

Olive oil

This is one of the best oils to use as substitute in cooking and baking. It has a rich fruity flavor that can either enhance flavor or blend into other stronger food flavors. This is also a popular item to perform liver cleanse- together with lemon juice.

Macadamia nut oil

Has the highest percentage of monounsaturated oil. It has the highest smoke point of all other unrefined oils in the market. Heat does not distort the structure easily, making it a stable fat and less likely to cause damage to the cells. Remember that heating the oils produces harmful byproducts like free radicals.

Coconut oil

Coconut oil is very healthy, especially if cold pressed and from organically grown coconut trees. It can be used for baking, stir frying and in salad dressings.

Foods with low glycemic index

Low glycemic index means that these foods do not cause rapid increase in the blood sugar levels. The list includes any meat or fat, because they do not contain any carbohydrates.

- Non starchy vegetables
- Fruits
- Rolled or steel-cut oatmeal, muesli and oat bran

- 100% stone ground grain and grain products
- Pasta, bulgur and barley
- Beans like black, navy, lima and pinto
- Legumes and lentils
- Corn, yam and sweet potato

Foods with medium glycemic index are consumed in moderate amounts.

- Pita bread, whole wheat rye and wheat bread
- Quick cooking oats
- Couscous and brown, basmati or wild rice

Whole grains

Whole grains are low glycemic index foods that are packed with minerals, vitamins, dietary fiber and antioxidants. The carbohydrates they contain are healthy, which do not cause dangerous sugar spikes. It actually helps in regulating carbohydrate metabolism and storage. It does not aggravate the fatty accumulations within the liver structure.

These are good replacement for high sugar processed food and snacks like white bread and breakfast cereals.

Good whole grain choices are spelt, barley, oats, brown or wild rice, rye and bulgur.

Bitter greens

These are liver detoxifying veggies. The list includes endive, watercress, arugula, parsley, dandelion and cilantro. These vegetables have astringent properties, which provide protection to the cells against damage from exposure to cigarette smoke, alcohol and pollution. At the same time, they revitalize and clean the gall bladder and the liver.

Proteins

Aim to eat about 1 to 2 servings of lean and healthy meats. Also, it is good for weight loss to snack on healthy and controlled portions of proteins when sudden pangs of hunger hit. Good sources are:

- Eggs from free-range and pastured chicken

- All seafood, either fresh or canned. However, stay away from deep fried or smoked seafood.
- Poultry, organically raised and free range
- Fresh lean meat
- Whey protein powder
- Legumes and raw nuts or seeds combination in the same meal or snack. Choices of legumes include chickpeas, beans and lentils. This combination is a first-0class protein source, which provides all the essential amino acids that the body needs. If nuts, seeds or legumes are taken alone, there is a great lack in nutrients, which does nothing to curb sugar cravings and stabilize blood sugar levels.

Healthy Snacking Guides

While losing weight and treating fatty liver with diet, there will times when you just have to snack. It's not falling off the wagon, as long as you snack on something healthy and in the right amounts.

- Mix one small can of seafood like mackerel, tuna, crabmeat or sardines with juice of half a lemon or a tablespoon of yogurt, then with some fresh herbs, roughly or finely chopped. Eat it as it is or use as dip for sliced veggie sticks.
- Make a protein-packed smoothie with almond milk or coconut milk with 3 tablespoons of berries.
- Snack on a handful of raw seeds or nuts or toss them with 1 medium-sized fruit. Sprinkle a pinch of salt if desired to enhance flavor.
- Raw vegetables like cucumber slices, zucchini, carrot and celery sticks, and broccoli florets. These may be eaten alone or dipped in healthy hummus, tahini or into some mashed fresh avocados.
- 1 to 2 medium-sized fruits, alone or with seeds, nuts or plain yogurt.
- One full glass of raw vegetable juice.
- Bean or avocado dip with raw vegetables or slightly steamed

cauliflower or broccoli florets.

Super foods

Yes, the body's detoxifier also needs to be detoxified every once in a while. Cruciferous vegetables like broccoli help in detoxifying the liver. Have at least a cup (1 serving) a day. The list includes:

- Collards, kale, Brussels sprouts, daikon radish and cabbage.
- Onions and garlic also detoxify the liver with their high sulfur content.

Vitamins and Minerals

Different minerals and vitamins help boost liver health, protecting against further damage and relives fatty deposits.

B vitamins

They help in detoxifying the liver, aiding in healing and prevention of further damage and complications. One of the important uses of B vitamins is that they help in breaking down cholesterol and bile in the liver.

Zinc

Zinc is known for its ability to speed up the process of healing in the body. This mineral also helps in neutralizing the damaging effects of free radicals. It boosts the immune system, helping it to strengthen and improve the protective and healing function. When the liver is compromised due to fatty deposits, a strong and healthy immune system gets a lot of the workload off the liver. This gives the liver a chance to heal itself.

Antioxidants

Antioxidants stop free radicals from damaging the cells. This is especially important during the recovery from a fatty liver. The excess fats metabolized release free radicals as by-products. hence, while the liver is recovering from the fat excess, it also releases harmful molecules into the body. That is when the action of antioxidants is most needed. This way, the liver can proceed with its healing, while the rest of the body is protected.

Choline

Choline is one of the important B vitamin in the body. It specifically helps in fat transport from the liver. By increasing the amount of choline in the body, more fats can be transported outside of the liver.

Foods rich in choline include beef liver, peanuts and egg yolks.

Vitamin E

Vitamin E helps in reducing the inflammation in the body, including in the liver. Though it does not directly affect fibrosis, vitamin E helps in the prevention of scar tissue formation. Inflammation causes the tissues of the liver to become fibrous and stiff (fibrosis). Over time, these fibrotic tissues will cause permanent impairment in the liver functioning. Vitamin E reduces inflammation in order to reduce the rate and amount of fibrotic tissues formed.

Vitamin C

Vitamin C has powerful antioxidant properties that have profound health benefits. A preliminary study found out that the combination of vitamin C and E has the potential to reverse fatty liver disease. More thorough study is still needed to determine the safety parameters and recommended dosages of this combination treatment.

Vitamin C in itself has protective properties. As an antioxidant, it protects the cells from free radical and toxin damage. When the liver is suffering from damage from fatty deposits and inflammatory reaction, vitamin C protects the damaged cells and healthy cells from further damage. This slows the progression of the disease, provides the liver tissues time to heal and prevents spread of damage.

Niacin

Niacin helps in reversing and eventual recovery of fatty liver by lowering the levels of triglycerides in the body. High triglyceride levels are one of the major risk factors for fatty liver. By lowering them, niacin keeps the liver from suffering further damage. This provides time for healing and recovery within the damaged liver structure.

Chapter 5 Herbs for a Healthier Liver

Herbs are rich in natural compounds that help heal the liver. Most are already being used to promote better liver health for centuries, which include the following:

Milk thistle

It has been used for centuries as an herbal remedy to protect the liver from toxic substances. The seed is known to help in the healing and restoration of damaged liver cells. Milk thistle is available in supplemental form. It contains active flavonoid complex that provides protection to the cells against damage from free radicals and from inflammation. The American Liver Society has even listed milk thistle as one of the foods that can restore the liver's normal structure and functioning.

Golden Seal

It is a powerful liver cleanser that helps in purifying the liver. It speeds up the removal of toxins and other harmful compounds from the liver. It can also help in restoring the liver to its normal functioning.

Green Tea

This contains powerful antioxidants. It facilitates the removal of the toxins from the liver and allows the liver to heal itself naturally. Green tea can be consumed safely on a daily basis, as tea.

Dandelion extract

The extract contains active compounds that help in cleansing the liver. It stimulate bile production. Toxins and fat cells are removed from the liver through the bile. The bile brings all these to the intestines fro excretion via the feces.

Soy protein

Studies have shown that consuming soy protein helps in reducing the rate and amount of fat that accumulates in the liver and the rest of the body. The soy proteins also help in restoring g the health, vitality and normal functioning of the liver cells. Sources include yogurt, tofu, soya beans and soy milk.

Flavonoids

These nutrients provide protection to the cells against damage. They also help in eliminating fat cells that cause inflammation and other problems in the liver and the rest of the body. Flavonoids are found in all colorful vegetables and fruits.

Burdock

Burdock plant is rich in vitamin B and E. These two vitamins help in repairing the liver and in restoring its full function.

Herbs to avoid

While herbs can help in restoring liver health, some contain compounds that may cause damage if the liver is already compromised.

Mistletoe

This good herb helps in calming the body. It also has antispasmodic effects. The extract is often used as natural herbal remedy for respiratory problems like cough and asthma. Mistletoe is also taken for its immune-boosting effects, which can help in speeding up liver recovery, however, if improperly taken, it can worsen an already compromised liver.

Yerba mate

If consumed in large amounts, it can increase the risk for liver cancer.

Peppermint and other products that contain menthol

This herb is used as liver detoxifiers, in small, controlled amounts. A damaged or compromised liver cannot tolerate large amounts of menthol. Oil forms of the herb are also too aggressive for a compromised liver to handle. It will cause very elevated levels of liver enzymes.

Valerian

This is toxic to the liver in large amounts.

Nutmeg

Contains the compound trimyristin, which is a saturated fat form that worsens fatty liver disease.

Pennyroyal

Contains compounds that are highly toxic to the cells in the liver and kidneys

Kava root

When taken as traditional tea, the active compounds are highly toxic to the liver. It may cause significant liver damage.

Sample Meal Plans

Whatever works for you is fine, as long as you keep within the basic rules (fruits and vegetables, no red meats, refined carbohydrates and unhealthy fats). Some swear by juicing and some by using olive oil. To help you in your way, here are a few suggestions.

Breakfast

This is the most important meal of the day. Jumpstart your day with a healthy amount of energy-giving foods that is safe for the liver.

Have skim milk with whole grain toast smeared with non-hydrogenated margarine. Better yet, use real butter. You would be surprised how much hydrogenated oils (trans fat) is present in margarine, no matter how "healthy" the label screams.

Aside from skim milk (fat "skimmed" from the surface), drink fresh citrus juices. The vitamin C boosts the body's energy for the day and at the same has antioxidants that protect cells from damage and inflammation.

Add fresh fruits like a medium-sized grapefruit or banana. Yogurt is also a good addition to the breakfast plate.

Coffee in the morning is also a good choice. Some research supports the healthy benefit of coffee on fatty liver. One study has even gone to illustrate that drinking 2 cups of coffee a day reduces scarring within the liver tissues and supports faster healing.

Lunch

Fill up on energy-boosting foods for the rest of the day. Have a sandwich of whole grain bread with white meats like turkey or chicken breast. You can also have canned tuna on whole rye bread. Avoid cheeses and marbled meats like corned beef. The more processing, the unhealthier it is.

To avoid palate boredom, vary. If you had toast for breakfast, have clear consommé or vegetable soup. It's best to make this from scratch, using fresh and whole ingredients. Homemade soups are more likely to be liver friendly than store-bought or restaurant made ones.

Tossed salads are also good lunch options. Mix some greens with beans, sprinkled with raw seeds or nuts. Drizzle healthy salad dressings like balsamic vinegar and other vinegar-based ones such as vinaigrettes.

Have a slice of fruit for dessert. It is naturally sweet but not the bad kind of sugar. Still, it's sugar so keep within the recommended daily amounts (not more than 2-3 servings).

Drink water infused with herbs or with a twist of lemon to increase metabolism.

Snack

To get you through the energy drain in the afternoons, snack healthy on salt-free nuts or graham crackers. Other good snack options are fruit slices and dark chocolate of good quality. Vegetable sticks are also great. For variety, dip in natural peanut butter (oil should be floating on top).

Dinner

You can eat a larger meal at dinner, but should still be within the recommended daily calorie allowance. Eat lean, low fat, healthy cuts of meat. Fish and skinless poultry are also good choices. It is best to leave off the meat sauce and gravies. Add a siding of vegetables, cooked in a healthy way. Baked, steamed, or roasted vegetables are fine, just not fried.

Add carbohydrates in the form of dinner roll. It should be made from whole grain like rye, or whole wheat. Potato is also good, but only a few times a week. Do not make it a daily part of the meal. Potato starch, in large amounts, can still contribute to fatty liver.

For dessert, a slice of fruit is good, or sugar-free jello. Avoid sugar substitutes can spell trouble so stay away from labeled "sugar free", unless it's Stevia- the only proven safe and healthy sugar substitute. No cakes, cookies and other desserts made from refined flour and white sugar.

Drink with water- infused or with a squeeze of lemon. Or you can also have skim milk for dinner.

As a general guide, follow these for a liver-friendly meal:

- Choose low fat foods
- Choose foods naturally low in fat

- No to artificial flavors- they contain high levels of salt, additives and refined carbohydrates
- Choose fresh and whole produce like organically grown vegetables and fruits
- Avoid eating in fast food chains- they have the most unhealthy foods ever
- Anything processed is bad
- No to soft drinks and sugary or salty snacks

Chapter 6 Natural Seven Day Liver Cleanse

Liver cleanse is the natural way in rejuvenating the liver and helping it restore its normal, proper functioning. Regular liver cleansing helps in minimizing the damaging effects of toxins and other harmful substances. This is also good to perform after a course of medication therapy, like after a short course of steroids or antibiotics. Medications can cause scarring and inflammation in the liver tissues. After a course, liver cleanse will remove much of the leftover toxins that may cause log term damage.

7-day Liver Cleanse

The simplest liver cleanse often involves taking lemon juice. Extract the juice from about half a dozen of lemons. Store it in an airtight container. Whenever you want or need to cleanse, get half tablespoon of the lemon juice and mix it to a glass of water, lukewarm. Drink on an empty stomach. Then take half glass of lemon juice after every meal. Do not add anything to the lemon juice, not even salt or sugar. Do this for 7 days for successful liver cleanse and restore it to its health.

What you Can do During the 7-day Liver Cleanse

Here's the daily activities in order to ensure proper 7-day liver cleanse and reap the maximum benefits.

Day 1

Totally change the food intake. Eat only fruits, whole grains and vegetables. They can be raw or cooked, but to get the best liver cleanse, eat them raw. Do not eat anything else that does not belong top this group of foods.

Expect that the energy levels will be low during this first, especially if the normal diet is rich in carbohydrates, particularly the white, refined ones. It is advisable to start the 7-day liver cleanse when there will not be too many activities required for the day. Better yet, do it on a Saturday, when there will be less work for the day.

Day 2 to 4

The next 3 days will be dedicated to a purely liquid diet. Liquids include fruit juices, herbal teas, vegetable juices and water- lots and lots of water. The aim of the 3-day liquid diet is to promote flushing.

Liquids are absorbed faster by the body. It also leaves very little residue when it comes to the digestive process. Hence, liquids are almost 100% absorbed and utilized, leaving little for fat storage.

By filling up on liquids, there is more liquid in the blood, which speeds up the excretion process via the kidneys. Simply put, the more liquid intake, the faster the kidneys and urinary bladder fill up, the faster the toxins are flushed out of the body.

By taking in fruits and vegetable juices, the antioxidants and fibers are better absorbed by the body. the fibers will mop up the free radicals and toxins in the body. They bind with these harmful chemicals and bring them out for excretion. The water helps to dilute the blood so that more blood will be brought to the kidneys to speed up elimination.

During these days, expect to feel tired most of the time- and cranky. The body will be depending on fat metabolism for energy, rather than from food intake. It will get better though, as the body starts to adjust top this new food intake pattern.

Day 5 to 6

At this point, start introducing solid foods back into the diet. it should be with raw vegetables and fruits, nothing else. After the purely liquid diet, gradually adding solid foods helps the body-and the digestive system- to revert into eating solids again.

It should be a gradual process, because otherwise, the digestive system will be overwhelmed by the digestive requirement of proteins and fats. Likely, cramps, bloating, nausea and vomiting will result. So take it slowly.

Day 7

This time, start eating cooked vegetables in addition to raw fruits and vegetables. This will prepare the body to adjust to the digestive enzymes released to digest cooked foods.

During the first 3 days of the liver cleanse, expect to feel out of sorts. The body is adjusting to the abrupt change of dietary intake. It is forced to depend on other energy sources like fat and protein metabolism. Also, expect low energy levels and emotional unrest like anger and having a short temper. The body is also adjusting to the sudden increase in toxins released and excreted from the body.

Benefits of Liver Cleanse

To keep your focus, here's what can be gained from the ordeal:

- Increased vitality, especially of the liver
- Reduction of disease symptoms. While fatty liver itself has no symptoms, the associated ones like high blood pressure and fatigue, jaundice and frequent headaches will be reduced.
- Improved liver function. The liver will now be back on track on its functions like fat metabolism and blood sugar regulation (via the hormone insulin)
- Weight loss. Notice that in 1 week, the calorie intake is severely reduced. The 1st week is crucial because this is when the most weight loss occurs. Hence, take advantage of the 7-day liver cleanse. You are hitting 2 birds with one stone- ridding the body of waste and jumpstarting weight loss.
- Improved skin characteristics. By ridding the body of wastes and toxins, the skin clears up. it would be surprising for some to know that dull, dry and problematic skin (e.g., prone to acne, etc.) stems from the accumulation of toxins in the skin layers.

Tips for Success

The liver cleanse is a tough week, no going around that. You may feel intense cravings, crankiness and anger, even depression. The body is abruptly deprived of all foods that it used to enjoy. Here's a few to help hurdle through the hardships that may hinder successful liver cleanse.

Cravings, low energy and irritability are the hardest to combat during the 1st 3 days of the liver cleanse. To help tide you over, keep liver-friendly snacks at hand. Have fresh vegetable and fruit slices readily available, already cut and portioned. Carrot sticks and apple slices in small containers should always be readily available should the craving become too intense. This way, you avoid inadvertently snacking on something that should be avoided, in the midst of intense, crazy cravings.

Do not eat every time the urge comes. Try to eat within the scheduled meals. Snacking too much will still defeat the purpose of a liver cleanse.

Keep hydrated. Water is very important in a liver cleanse, as it will be the main driving force for excretion. Water will cause the toxins to be flushed out of the body. drinking water will also help in achieving a feeling of fullness, the better to combat the hunger pangs.

Eat (or drink) lots of fiber. More fibers mean more of this stuff that absorbs and binds the toxins for easy excretion. fibers also help in feeling full longer.

Other foods that cleanse the liver

Artichokes

Artichokes increases bile production. More toxins are excreted if there is a lot of bile that can bind them. Bile then brings these toxins to the intestines for excretion. Also, other vegetables like leafy greens, chicory and endive also help in stimulating bile production for liver cleansing.

Garlic and onions

According to Disabled World, allicin compound in onions and garlic contain sulfur that promotes detoxification of the liver. Best way to take it is by crushing or chopping them finely. Add them raw to food or at the end of the cooking process to preserve the healing properties.

Chapter 7 Prevention

Prevention is much easier than treatment. Fatty liver generally goes away on its own, but also

Maintain ideal body weight

The ideal body weight, measured in BMI (body mass index) should be between 18 and 24.5. For every increase, risk is also increased, not only for fatty liver but for other chronic health problems, too.

If the present body weight is above the ideal, lose weight. Do so safely. Aim to lose 1 kilogram or 1 to 2 pounds each week. Losing a lot in a short time is actually bad for the body. Chronic illnesses may be aggravated or new ones may develop.

Aim for good lipid profile

Keep the lipoproteins in the right and healthy balance. Aim for low LDL and triglycerides, and high HDL levels.

Keep off too much alcohol consumption

Alcohol consumption is a major factor in fatty liver development. Stay within the recommended amount of daily intake. a recent study showed that drinking 1 glass of wine per day could actually decrease the risk for developing nonalcoholic fatty liver disease. Results showed that the risk is reduced by half, compared to people who did not take any amount of wine in a day.

Beer and liquor, according to the same study, do not provide any protection. It was found out that drinking 1 ounce of liquor or 12 ounces of beer increases the risk for NASH (nonalcoholic steatohepatitis).

Conclusion

Thank you again for downloading this book!

I hope this book was able to help you to learn more about curing fatty liver and the wonders of alternative treatments.

At the same time I hope that this book was able to help you better understand your role in curing your own fatty liver, and that having a healthy lifestyle that includes the right diet and ample amount of exercise are very important to cure and prevent fatty liver.

I hope this book served as a guide for healthier living.

Finally, if you enjoyed this book, please take the time to share your thoughts and post a review on Amazon. We do our best to reach out to readers and provide the best value we can. Your positive review will help us achieve that. It'd be greatly appreciated!

Thank you and good luck!